Latifa MTIBAA
Wiem KOUKI
Boutheina JEMLI

Toxoplasmosis in pregnant women

Latifa MTIBAA
Wiem KOUKI
Boutheina JEMLI

Toxoplasmosis in pregnant women

Contribution of serological diagnosis

ScienciaScripts

Imprint

Any brand names and product names mentioned in this book are subject to trademark, brand or patent protection and are trademarks or registered trademarks of their respective holders. The use of brand names, product names, common names, trade names, product descriptions etc. even without a particular marking in this work is in no way to be construed to mean that such names may be regarded as unrestricted in respect of trademark and brand protection legislation and could thus be used by anyone.

Cover image: www.ingimage.com

This book is a translation from the original published under ISBN 978-620-6-71860-4.

Publisher:
Sciencia Scripts
is a trademark of
Dodo Books Indian Ocean Ltd. and OmniScriptum S.R.L publishing group

120 High Road, East Finchley, London, N2 9ED, United Kingdom
Str. Armeneasca 28/1, office 1, Chisinau MD-2012, Republic of Moldova, Europe
Printed at: see last page
ISBN: 978-620-8-23804-9

List of abbreviations

Ac: antibody

ECLIA: Electro-chimiluminescence immunoassay

ELISA: Enzyme-Linked Immunosorbent **Assay**

GRA 1: Dense granule proteins 1

GRA 7: Dense granule proteins 7

GRA 8: Dense granule proteins 8

HMPIT: Hôpital Militaire Principal d'Instruction de Tunis (Tunis Main Military Instruction Hospital)

IFI: indirect immunofluorescence

IgA: immunoglobulin **A**

IgG: immunoglobulin G

IgM: immunoglobulin M

MIC 3: Micronème 3

Pe: proportion of a random agreement

Po: proportion of agreement observed

SAG 1: *Surface Antigen* 1

SAG 2: *Surface Antigen* 2

TMB: tetramethylbenzidine

Contents

Introduction

<u>Introduction</u>

Certain infectious diseases cause unexplained abortions in pregnant women and malformations in newborn babies. Toxoplasmosis is one such disease that poses a global health problem [1]. In Tunisia, prevalence is estimated at between 47% and 58% in 2018, and varies significantly with age (52% at age 20 and 70% at age 30) [2].

Toxoplasmosis is a cosmopolitan zoonosis caused by an obligate intracellular parasite, *Toxoplasma gondii*, which occurs in various forms: tachyzoite, bradyzoite and oocyst [3]. It can be transmitted by various routes: ingestion, organ transplantation, blood transfusion and transplacental transmission [4].

There are three clinical entities: acquired postnatal toxoplasmosis in the immunocompetent subject (the mild form), toxoplasmosis in the immunocompromised subject (the severe form) and congenital toxoplasmosis. Congenital toxoplasmosis results from transmission of the parasite from mother to fetus after a primary maternal infection. Toxoplasmas cross the placenta and infect the fetus, resulting in abortion, fetal death in utero or severe malformations with central nervous system damage. These severe forms are mainly observed in the case of seroconversions early in pregnancy, due to the immaturity of the fetal immune system; as the term of the mother's infection advances, the risk of severe forms diminishes in favour of benign or latent forms [5].

This primary infection produces antibodies of various isotypes (immunoglobulin M (IgM), immunoglobulin G (IgG), immunoglobulin A (IgA)) specifically directed against parasite antigens [6]. It is therefore essential to have several discriminating serological techniques to detect any seroconversion in pregnant women, and to date the infection, IgM being characteristic of the acute phase and IgG revealing an older infection. IgG avidity tests can also be used to determine the date of infection [7]. These include the Dye Test, indirect immunofluorescence (IFI), electrochemiluminescence (ECLIA) and Enzyme-Linked Immunosorbent Assay (ELISA) [4]. However, day-to-day interpretation is fraught with difficulties, the most common of which relate to the non-standardization of reagents, which can lead to erroneous interpretations or discrepancies in status, given that the various serological interpretation strategies are based on combining the results of several tests [8] . For this reason, comparable measures must be taken as part of good medical practice to ensure the best possible interpretation.

The aim of our study is to:

-        Compare anti-Toxoplasma *gondii* serology (IgG) results in pregnant women using three techniques:
→   ECLIA (Elecsys® Toxo IgG)
→   ELISA (Platelia™ Testline TOXO IgG) and (Platelia™ Toxo IgG)
→   And WESTERN BLOT (Blot-line *Toxoplasma* IgG).

Materials and methods

<u>Hardware</u>

1.   Study description:

1.1. Type of study :

- This is a cross-sectional study carried out in the Parasitology-Mycology laboratory of the Hôpital militaire principal d'instruction de Tunis between January 23, 2023 and April 15, 2023.

1.2 Study population

- The study population consisted of 53 pregnant women referred to the Parasitology-Mycology laboratory for toxoplasmosis serology.

1.2.1   Inclusion criteria:

- The women included in this study are pregnant and immunized with a serological profile (IgG+ and IgM-).

1.2.2   Exclusion criteria :

- Non-pregnant women of childbearing age.
- Pregnant women with serological profiles (IgG- and IgM+) or (IgG+ and IgM+) or (IgG- and IgM-).

2.   Materials used :

2.1. Consumables

Single-use tubes.

- Single-use gloves.

- End caps.

- Adjustable or fixed pipettes, capable of measuring and delivering 10 µl to 100 µl, 1 ml, 2 ml.

- Rack.

 - Absorbent paper.

- Stopwatch.

- Transparent adhesive film.

2.2. Reagents used

2.2.1. Elecsys® Toxo IgG (Appendix1)

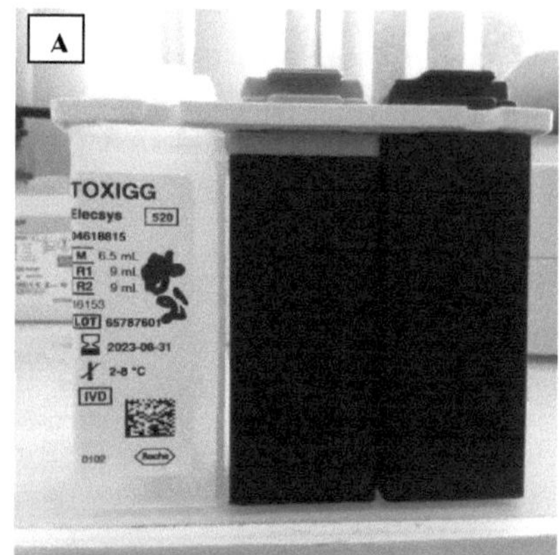
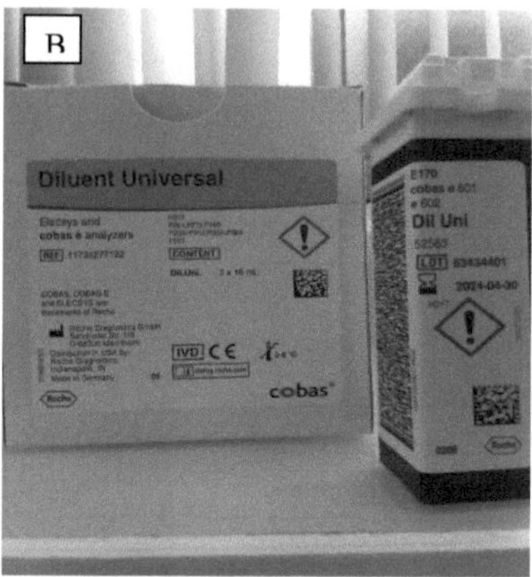

Figure 1A: Reagent rackpack (M, R1, R2) B: Sample diluent

(Parasitology Laboratory, HMPIT)

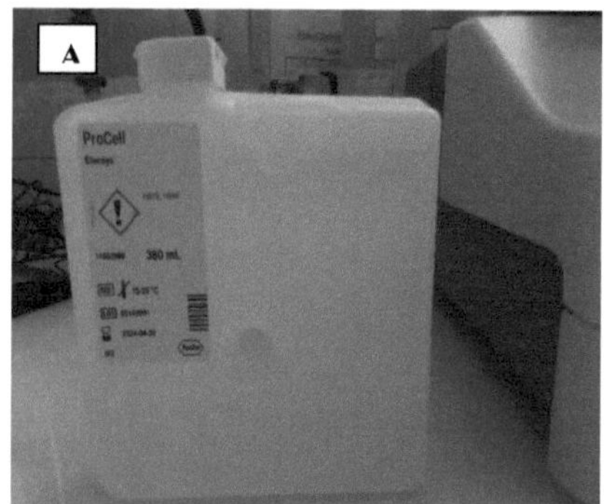
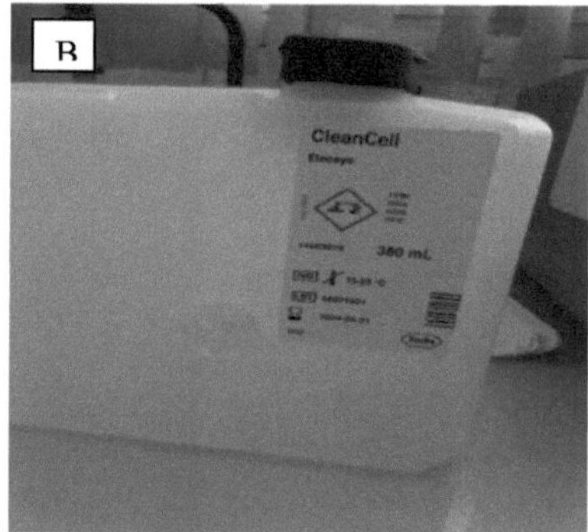

Figure 2A: ProCell buffer system; B: ClenCell wash solution for measuring cell

(Parasitology Laboratory, HMPIT)

2.2.2. Platelia TM Testline TOXO IgG kit (Appendix 2)

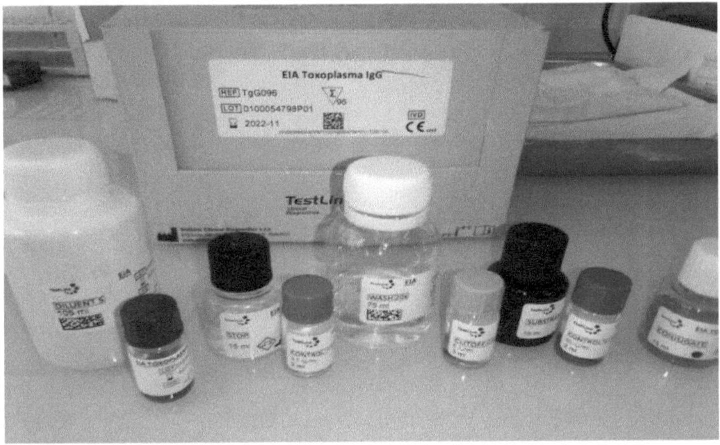

Figure 3 Platelia TM Testline TOXO IgG reagents

(Parasitology Laboratory, HMPIT)

2.2.3. *Toxoplasma* IgG Blot-line kit (Appendix 3)

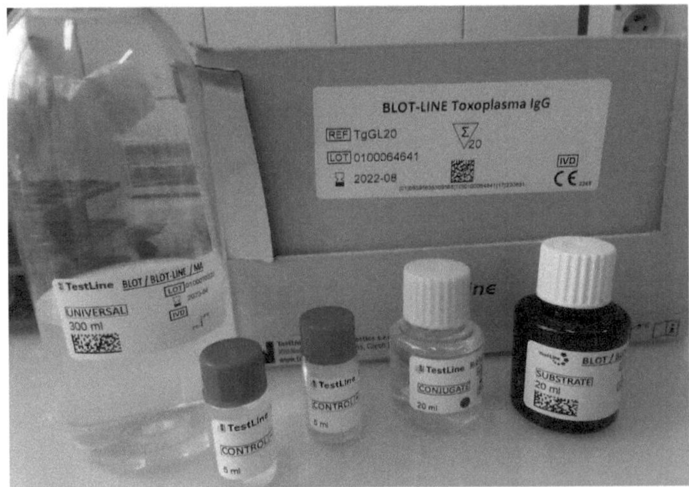

Figure 4*Toxoplasma* IgG Blot-line reagents

(Parasitology Laboratory, HMPIT)

2.2.4. Platelia kit™ Biorad TOXO IgG (Appendix 4)

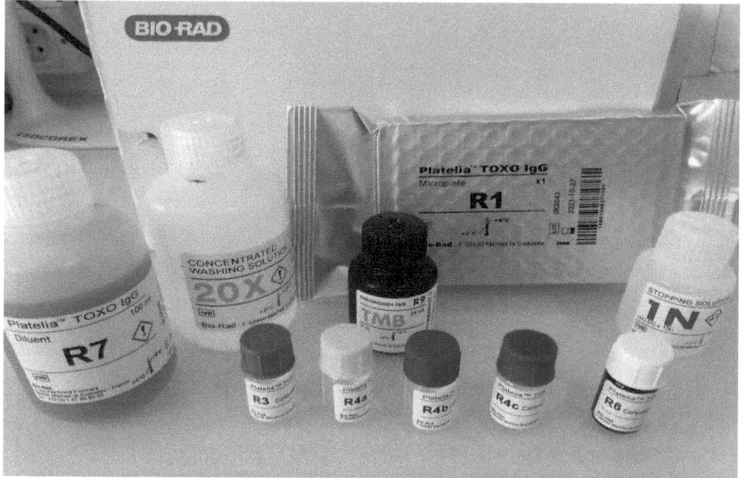

Figure 5: Platelia TM Biorad TOXO IgG reagents

(Parasitology Laboratory, HMPIT)

2.3. Equipment

*Juicer

*Spectrophotometer

*Vacuum cleaner

*Cobas e 411

*incubator

*Designer

<u>Methods</u>

1.   Study methodology :

We studied the IgG titer in 53 sera from pregnant women initially tested by ECLIA (Elecsys® Toxo IgG), subdivided into three groups according to IgG levels: one group with levels ranging from 30 to 300 IU/ml, the second from 300 to 1000 IU/ml and the last above 1000 IU/ml. These sera were then re-tested by ELISA (Platelia™ Biorad), ELISA (Platelia™ Testline) and Blot-line *Toxoplasma* IgG.

2.   Data collection :

The data collection form was used to gather the various data needed to compare our results with those of the literature, including the parameters required for our work: **age, number of pregnancies (gestational age), parity, gestational age of the current pregnancy** (Appendix 5).

3.   Blood sampling :

Blood is drawn from the superficial vein in the elbow, after disinfecting the site and applying a tourniquet. The blood is then collected in dry tubes.

4.   Techniques used for IgG determination

The blood sample is centrifuged at 3,500 rpm for 9 minutes. After centrifugation, the serum is separated and used for the serological assay.

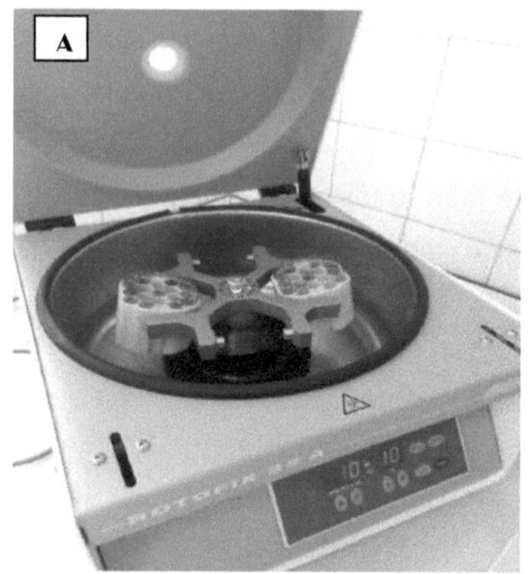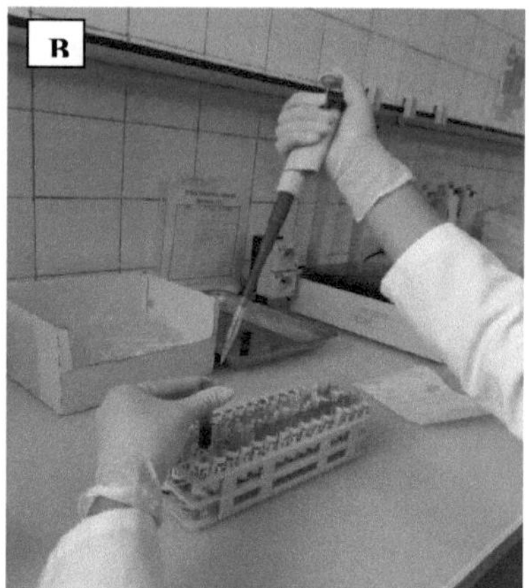

Figure 6A: Centrifugation of serological tubes; B: Blood separation

(Parasitology Laboratory, HMPIT)

4.1 ECLIA: Electro-Chemi-luminescent-immuno-assay :

This technique was carried out on the Cobas e 411 automated system (Figure 7), enabling IgG to be titrated against a standard curve.

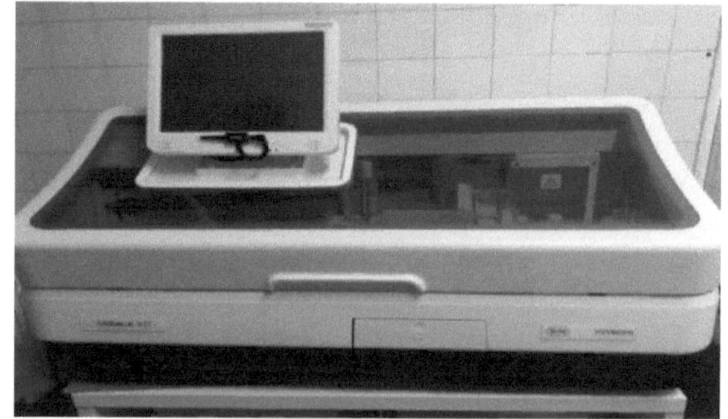

Figure 7COBASe411 controller

(Parasitology Laboratory, HMPIT)

4.1.1 Sandwich" principle :

▪ 1st incubation: 10 µL of sample are placed in the presence of biotinylated *T. gondii-specific* recombinant antigen and ruthenium-labeled T. *gondii-specific* recombinant antigen. A **"sandwich"** is formed.

▪ 2nd incubation: streptavidin-coated microparticles are added to the reaction cuvette. The immune complex is bound to the solid phase by a streptavidin-biotin bond.

▪ The reaction mixture is drawn into the measuring cell, where the microparticles are held at the electrode surface by a magnet. The free fraction is removed by passing ProCell or ProCell M. A potential difference applied to the electrode triggers the production of luminescence, which is measured by a photomultiplier.

▪ Results are obtained using a calibration curve and expressed in IU/ml. This is generated specifically for the analyzer used by a 2-point calibration and a reference curve stored in the -reagent's barcode label or -ecodebar **(Figure 8) (appendix 1)**

Total durati on of analy tical cycle: 18 minut es.

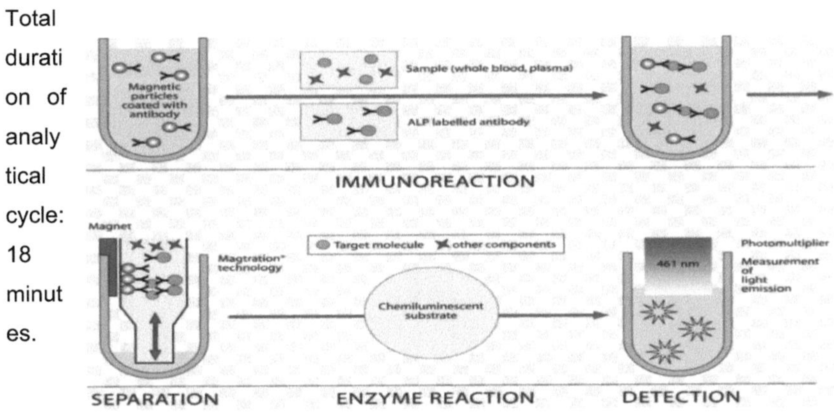

Figure 8: Schematic diagram of the ECLIA reaction principle

(https://www.freepng.fr/png-69juff/)

4.1.2. Interpreting the results :

Table I Interpretation of ECLIA results

Antibody titre	Interpretation
<1 IU/ml	Negative
1<x <30 IU/ml	Doubtful to do again after 3 weeks
≥30 IU/ml	Positive

4.2. ELISA: (Enzyme-Linked ImmunoSorbent Assay): Indirect method.

4.2.1. Principle of the ELISA technique

. The principle of this enzyme immunoassay technique is to bring maternal antibodies into contact with specific antigens. The resulting complexes are then detected by the addition of a labeled anti-antibody conjugate - an animal immunoglobulin fraction - to human IgG conjugated with horseradish peroxidase. Peroxidase activity is determined in the assay by a substrate containing TMB. Positivity is indicated when the blue color appears after the stop solution has been added, and the blue color changes to yellow. The intensity of the yellow color is measured by a photometer at 450 nm, and is proportional to the concentration of specific IgG antibodies in the sample (figure 9) (appendix 2 and 3).

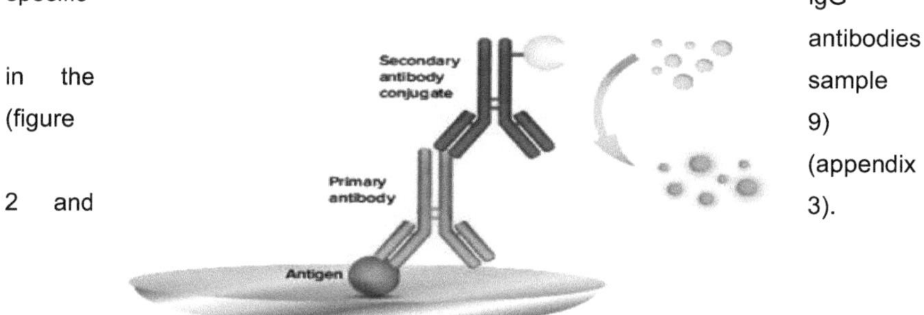

Figure 9 Schematic diagram of the ELISA reaction principle: Indirect ELISA

(https://fr.moleculardevices.com/applications/enzyme-linked-immunosorbent-assay-elisa#gref)

4.2.2. Interpretation of results (Platelia™ Testline semi-quantitative method)

Table II Interpretation of PlateliaTM Testline results (semi-quantitative method)

Index	Interpretation
<0.9	Negative
0.9<x <1.1	Doubtful
≥1.1	Positive

4.2.3. Interpretation of results (Platelia™ Biorad quantitative method)

Table III Interpretation of Platelia TM Biorad results (quantitative method)

Antibody titre	Interpretation
<6IU/ml	Negative
6<x<9 IU/ml	Doubtful
≥9 IU/ml	Positive

4.3. Blot-line *Toxoplasma* IgG

4.3.1. Principle :

The BLOT-LINE kit enables the detection of specific IgG antibodies against recombinant *Toxoplasma gondii* antigens in human serum or plasma.

Highly purified, recombinant antigens are transferred to a nitrocellulose membrane attached to a plastic buffer. In the first reaction step, individual strips are incubated with the sample under test, and specific antibodies (if present in the sample) bind to the corresponding commercial antigens on the strip. After washing, the strips are then incubated with a conjugate and visualized using a substrate solution. To check the validity of the tests, the strips include a conjugated control strip and a control strip indicating the kit's functionality and sensitivity (appendix 3).

4.3.2. Diagram of Blot-line *Toxoplasma* IgG strips

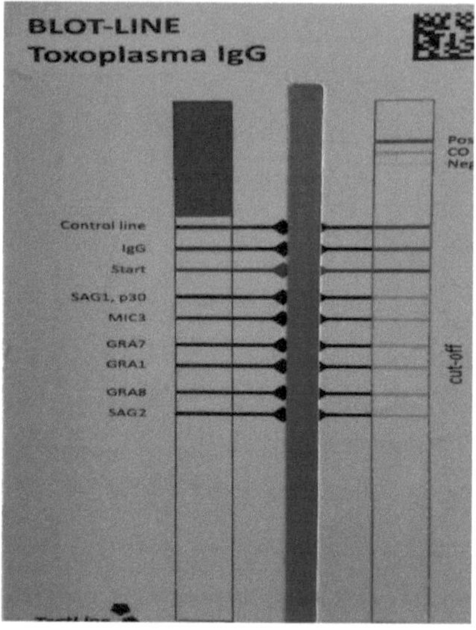

Figure 10 Blot-line Toxoplasma IgG strips

(Parasitology Laboratory, HMPIT)

16

4.3.3. Characteristics of each antigenic band expressed by *Toxoplasma gondii* :

Table IV<u>Characteristics of antigens expressed by *Toxoplasma gondii*</u>

Antigen	Description
SAG 1	p30; a highly immunogenic and antigenic surface antigen involved in the activation of the tachyzoite immune response during the acute phase of toxoplasmosis; a good serological marker for antibodies against *T. gondii* in the acute and chronic phase of infection; high titers of IgG, IgM and IgA.
MIC 3	p90; strong adhesion and is one of the leading vaccine candidates. It is a 90 kDa dimeric, cysteine-rich protein. It is expressed as tachyzoites, bradyzoites and sporozoites and has excellent immune properties.
GRA 1	p24; a highly immunogenic protein whose reactivity is to a large extent in the chronic phase of the disease.
GRA 7	p29; expressed in all infectious forms of toxoplasma. It provokes a strong antibody response in the acute phase of infection. It is considered an important diagnostic tool, adapted to the chronic phase of infection.
GRA 8	p35; highly immunogenic protein, more suitable for the acute phase than the chronic phase.
SAG 2	p22; a major surface protein known as a ligand. Effective for the detection of IgG antibodies in patients with acute toxoplasmosis.

Table V:<u>Interpretation of Blot-line results</u>

Specific antigen bands	Evaluation
At least one positive band	Positive
A dubious strip	Doubtful
No positive band	Negative

5.   Data recording and statistical analysis :

Data entry was performed using Microsoft Office Excel 2007 and SPSS version 22.0. The correlation coefficient between techniques was calculated using Cohen's kappa test.

5.1. Cohen's kappa coefficient: designed to measure agreement between two categorical variables, is defined by :

$$K = \frac{Po - Pe}{1 - Pe}$$

With

 K: Cohen's coefficient

Po: proportion of agreement observed

Pe: proportion of a random agreement

5.2. Interpretation :

Table VI<u>Interpretation of Cohen's coefficient</u>

K	Interpretation
<0	Disagreement
0 - 0.2	Very weak agreement
0.21_0.4	Weak agreement
0.41_0.6	Moderate agreement
0.61_0.8	Strong agreement
0.8_1	An almost perfect match

6. Ethical considerations :

The overall rules of confidentiality and patient data protection were taken into consideration during this work. All pregnant women are questioned, and their anonymity is respected during data analysis.

Results

<u>Results</u>

1. Age distribution of patients :

To determine the age distribution of the study population, we grouped them into 5-year age brackets. The results are shown in the following histogram:

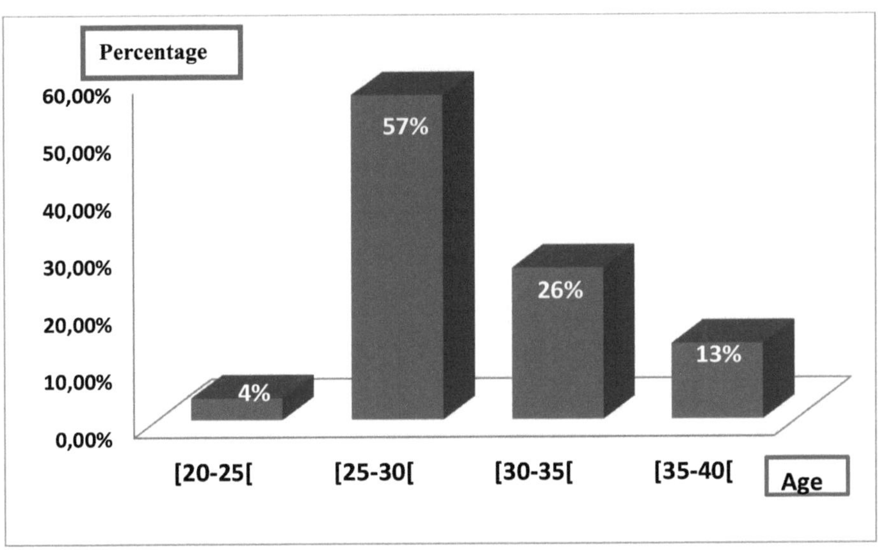

Figure 11 Age distribution of study population

According to the previous figure, the majority of pregnant women included in our +study are aged [25-30[years with a percentage of (57%). The mean age of our patients was 29 ± 3.9 years, with extremes of 22 and 40 years.

2. <u>Distribution of patients according to gestational age :</u>

Analysis of the gestational outcomes of the study population shows that the majority of pregnant women consulted the laboratory during their first pregnancies (72%).

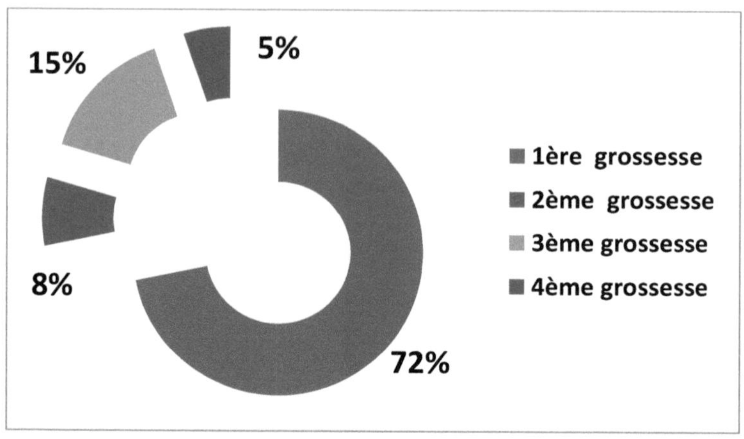

Figure 12 Distribution of patients according to gestational age

3.   Patient distribution by parity

Pregnancies older than 20 weeks of amenorrhea were considered. Our results show that 51% of pregnant women who presented for toxoplasmosis serology were primiparous.

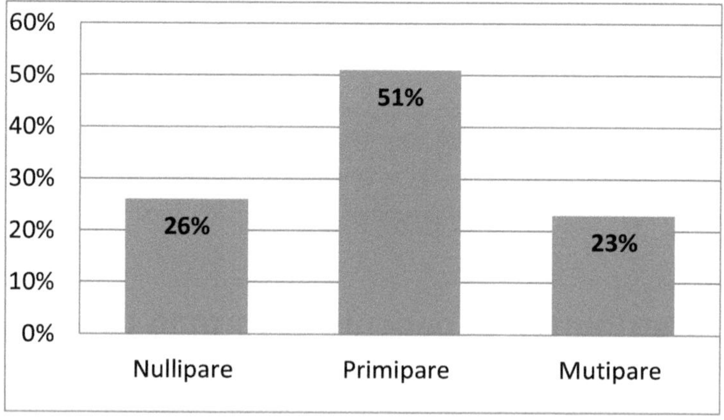

Figure 13 Distribution of patients by parity

4. <u>Distribution of patients by gestational age:</u>

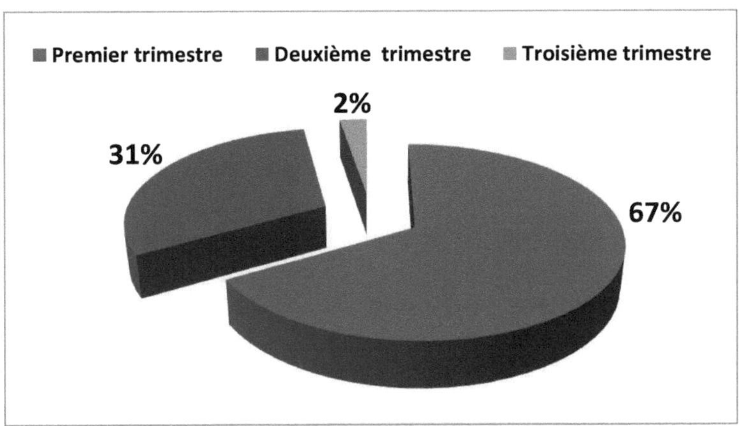

Figure 14: Distribution of patients by gestational age

The previous figure shows that 67% of patients undergoing toxoplasmosis testing were pregnant in the first trimester.

5. <u>Comparison between ECLIA (Elecsys® Toxo IgG) and ELISA (Platelia™ Biorad TOXO IgG)</u>

We subdivided the 53 sera from pregnant women into three groups according to IgG levels: G1 group with levels ranging from 30 to 300 IU/ml, G2 group with levels ranging from 300 to 1000 IU/ml and G3 group with levels above 1000 IU/ml. All the values found in the sera studied by the two techniques were above the positivity threshold, showing total concordance (P=1). We have tried to deduce a multiplication coefficient between the two techniques used. We note that, for our sample of sera studied, the values found by the ECLIA method (Elecsys® Toxo IgG) are higher than those found by ELISA (Platelia™ Biorad TOXO IgG).

Table VII Comparison between ECLIA (Elecsys Toxo IgG) and ELISA (Platelia TM Biorad TOXO IgG)

Number of sera studied	IgG titer By ECLIA in the study group	Average securities (ECLIA)	Title average (ELISA)	Multiplication coefficient
17	G1 [30 ; 300 IU/ml [	139	73	2
19	G2 [300;1000 IU/ml [	460	154	3
17	G3 ≥1000 IU/ml	1770	203	9

6.   <u>Comparison between ECLIA (Elecsys® Toxo IgG) and semi-quantitative ELISA (Platelia™ Testline TOXO IgG)</u>

All the values found in the sera studied by the two techniques were above the positivity threshold, showing total concordance (P=1).

Table VIII Comparison between ECLIA (Elecsys Toxo IgG) and ELISA (Platelia TM Testline TOXO IgG)

Number of sera studied	IgG titer By ECLIA in the study group	Average titles using the ECLIA technique	Average index IP
17	G1 [30 ; 300 IU/ml [	139	2,5
19	G2 [300;1000 IU/ml [	460	3,5
17	G3 ≥1000 IU/ml	1770	3,8

7. <u>Comparison between ECLIA (Elecsys® Toxo IgG) and Blot-line *Toxoplasma* IgG</u>

The table below shows one doubtful case out of eleven positive by the Blot-line technique, while all twelve cases are above the positivity threshold, indicating almost perfect agreement (P= 0.947).

Table IX Comparison between ECLIA and Blot-line *Toxoplasma* IgG

Syslab	1078	1527	1452	1741	762	1762	1644	1233	508	2019	1600	662
SAG 1	Dt	+	+	Dt	+	+	+	+	+	+	+	+
MIC 3	-	+	+	Dt	+	+	+	+	+	+	+	+
GRA7	-	-	+	Dt	+	-	+	+	+	+	Dt	+
GRA1	-	-	+	+	Dt	-	Dt	-	+	Dt	+	+
GRA8	Dt	-	Dt	Dt	+	+	+	+	+	+	dt	+
SAG2	-	-	-	-	-	-	-	-	-	-	-	-
+ / -	Dt	+	+	+	+	+	+	+	+	+	+	+
ECLIA IgG titre (IU/ml)	39	61	217	286	320	421	646	948	1168	1224	3057	4277

Dt: doubtful

Discussion

<u>Discussion</u>

Diagnosis of toxoplasmosis relies mainly on serological tests developed to detect antibodies (Ac) directed against antigens. The use of sensitive, reproducible serological tests, increasingly purified antigens and the demonstration of specific antibodies belonging to different isotypes, have solved most of the diagnostic problems of newly-acquired toxoplasmosis in immunocompetent patients.

Several manufacturers supply commercial tests for the determination and quantification of IgG, with generally good performance. The main shortcoming of these tests is the poor standardization of results between marketed techniques, due to variations in antigen quality from one kit to another. For this reason, we conducted our study with the aim of comparing commercially available techniques for the detection of *anti-Toxoplasma gondii* IgG in pregnant women.

The patients who participated ranged in age from 22 to 40 years, with an average age of 29 ± 3.9 years. Our study shows a predominance of pregnant women aged 25-30 years (57%), followed by those aged 30-35 years (26%). Our results are similar to those observed in a study by Christian Maucler Pamatika *et al* in the Central African Republic in 2020 [9], who reported an average age of pregnant women of 25 ± 6 years (with extremes of 16 and 40 years). They found that the population aged between 20 and 34 was the most represented (68%). The same finding was made by BELAID Amani *et al* in the Biskra region in 2022, where a large proportion of their included patients (61%) were women aged between 25 and 35 [10]. In fact, these age groups are considered to be the most active period in terms of childbearing and therefore correspond to the peak of gynecological consultations, hence the high frequency of visits to analysis laboratories by these age groups for toxoplasmosis serology.

Most requests for toxoplasmosis serology tests are made during the first pregnancy (72% of cases), followed by 15% during the third pregnancy. Results found in a study in Tizi-Ouzou by FERSAOUI Dehbia (2022) indicate that the percentage of women studied is close, with 56% of women being primigravida [11]. This test should be requested during the first pregnancy to determine the serological profile of the pregnant woman and avoid any complications.

According to the results obtained, most of our patients are primiparous (51%), although nulliparous women are also well represented (26%). These results concur with those of HAMMACI Lynda et *al* in TIZI OUZOU in 2020, whose study showed a predominance of primiparous women, with a frequency evaluated at 54.62% [12]. On the other hand, our study revealed a result contrary to those reported by Mariam HAMAICHAT (2020) in Guelmim, where around one-third of women were primiparous, and two-thirds were multiparous [13]. The predominance of primiparous women and the decrease in multiparous women are explained by good pregnancy monitoring.

Our study shows that most requests for toxoplasmosis serology were made in the first trimester (67%), followed by 31% in the second trimester. Other studies carried out in Algeria by FERSAOUI Dehbia (2022) et *al* found that 38% were in the first trimester of pregnancy and 34% in the second trimester [11]. In contrast to our results, a Moroccan study by Mustapha AKOURIM *et al* in 2016 observed that 26.23% of pregnant women attended the first consultation during the first trimester of gestational age, 36.72% during the second trimester and 37.05%during the third trimester [14].

The predominance of test requests during the first trimester is explained by the good skills of doctors, who request this serology as early as possible in the pregnancy. Regarding the availability of serological tests in the second and third trimesters, pregnant women delay their serological tests, probably due to lack of health education and low economic status. We note that, for our sample of sera studied, the values found by ECLIA and ELISA are above the positivity threshold, showing total concordance (p=1).

Villard *et al* (2016) reported a specificity of 100% and a sensitivity of 97.2% for the Platelia Toxo Biorad kit [15]. Robert-Gangneux in a study carried out in France (2021), showed a specificity of 99.6% and a sensitivity of 98.6% for the ECLIA technique [16]. On the other hand, the results obtained in our study by the ECLIA method are higher than those obtained by ELISA. The multiplication factors for

ECLIA vs ELISA results are 2 ,3 and 9 for IgG titers [30 ; 300 IU/ml [, [300 ;1000 IU/ml [and ≥1000 IU/ml respectively.

This difference can be explained by the difference in antigens used, as the early humoral immune response is first directed against parasite membrane antigens and then against cytoplasmic antigens once the immune response has matured. As a result, techniques using membrane antigens detect anti-toxoplasmic IgG earlier than those using cytoplasmic antigens. This early detection results in a time lag in the evolution of antibodies. Direct comparison of these two techniques is difficult, given the heterogeneity of detection thresholds. Expressing results in UI/ml tends to standardize them, but identical titres cannot be obtained with different antigens. Charlotte Martin found the same result, knowing that Platelia (Biorad) uses antigens relatively close to those of Vidas, giving a similar evolution of detected antibodies, Charlotte concluded that there was a 15-day lag between the IgG kinetic curves of AxSYM (Abbot) and Vidas® (Biomérieux). AxSYM ® (Abbott) uses membrane antigens like ECLIA [6].

In the comparison between ECLIA (Elecsys® Toxo IgG) and semi-quantitative ELISA (Platelia™ Testline TOXO IgG), all the values found in the sera studied were above the positivity threshold, showing complete agreement (P=1). This agreement can be explained by the high sensitivity of the two techniques. These results concur with those of Aref Teimouri, who showed 98% agreement [17].Concerning the comparison between ECLIA and Blot-line Toxo IgG, we showed almost perfect agreement (P= 0.947) between the two techniques.

Only one case was doubtful by Blot-line and positive by ECLIA, with a weakly positive IgG level of 39 IU/ml. This discrepancy can be explained by the positivity threshold (30 IU/ml), which is very close to the value found.

Robert-Gangneux (2021) reported in a systematic review of studies evaluating the performance of marketed kits for the detection of *anti-Toxoplasma* IgG a specificity of 99.6% and a sensitivity of 98.6% for the ECLIA technique [16]. The latter showed in this review an average sensitivity ranging from 89.7% to 100% and a specificity ranging from 91.3% to 100% for several techniques including western blot, which explains this good inter-technique agreement [16]. With regard to bands, the SAG 1 band, which corresponds to a high IgG titer, appeared in sera with a high IgG titer (n=10; 83%). In a study carried out in Brittany by Sarah Dion in 2019, she showed that almost 100% of patients expressed antibodies directed against SAG1 [18]. The SAG2 band never appeared in the sera studied, as it corresponds to an acute infection. The longer the infection, the more the MIC 3 specific band appears, as the micronemes involved in the invasion stage are exposed to the immune system secondarily to SAG.

Conclusion and outlook

<u>Conclusion and outlook</u>

Toxoplasmosis is one of the most common diseases affecting pregnant women, with serious or even fatal consequences in the event of seroconversion. Anti-toxoplasmic antibodies are markers of infection and form the basis of toxoplasmosis screening and monitoring.

Diagnosis of toxoplasma seroconversion is not always straightforward. It requires a good understanding of the kinetic variability of antibodies produced to date maternal contamination, with a view to early and appropriate treatment.

We conducted a cross-sectional study in the Parasitology-Mycology laboratory of the Hôpital militaire principal d'instruction de Tunis between January 23, 2023 and April 15, 2023. We studied IgG titres in 53 sera from pregnant women, with the aim of comparing several serological techniques for the detection of antitoxoplasmic IgG: quantitative ELISA (Platelia Toxo), semi-quantitative ELISA (Platelia™ Testline TOXO IgG), ECLIA (Elecsys® Toxo IgG) and Western Blot (Blot-line *Toxoplasma* IgG).

The mean age of our patients was 29 ± 3.9 years. Serologies were requested during their first pregnancies (72%), in primiparous women (51%) and in 67% during the first trimester. We found that quantitative and semi-quantitative ELISA and ECLIA were in complete agreement (P=1) in terms of positivity, but showed a difference in IgG titres due to shifting kinetic curves. On the other hand, an almost perfect agreement (P= 0.947) was found when comparing ECLIA and Western blot, given the presence of a doubtful case by Western blot with an IgG level of 39 IU/ml close to the positivity threshold (30 IU/ml) of ECLIA.

In the future, screening for toxoplasmosis could be modified. It would be advisable to set up a serological surveillance program during pregnancy as a first step towards preventing toxoplasmosis. It is also important to improve diagnostic techniques and standardize the toxoplasma antigens used in commercial kits.

References

References

[1]: Fanigliulo D, Marchi S, Montomoli E, Trombetta CM. Toxoplasma gondii in women of childbearing age and during pregnancy: a seroprevalence study in central and southern Italy from 2013 to 2017. Can J Public Health. 2019;110(3):398-402

[2]: Programme conjoint en santé maternelle et néonatale. Essential care baskets in maternal and newborn health. December 2018.

[3] Robert-Gangneux F, Dion S. Toxoplasmosis in pregnant women. J Pediatr Puéric. 2020;33:209-220.

[4] : HAS. Diagnosis biologique de la toxoplasmose acquise du sujet immunocompétent (dont la femme enceinte), la toxoplasmose congénitale (diagnostic pré- et postnatal) et la toxoplasmose oculaire. Has Haute Autorité De Santé. 2017.

[5]: Association française des enseignants et praticiens hospitaliers titulaires de parasitologie et mycologie médicales. Parasitoses et mycoses: Réussir les ECNi. Elsevier Masson. 2019.

[6] : Martin C. Toxoplasmosis serology: comparison of two techniques: Platelia microplate (biorad) and automate liaison (DIASORIN); study of avidity of anti-toxoplasmic IgG. Ann Biol Clin (Paris). 2006;64(3):245-250.

[7]: Gynaecology Obstetrics Fertility and Senology. Toxoplasmosis during pregnancy: current proposal for practical management. Elsevier Masson France. 2019.

[8]: Difficulties in interpreting toxoplasmosis serology. Rev Francoph Lab. 2022;545:33-39.

[9]: Pamatika CM, Sembene N, Mbeko-Simaleko M, Nembi G, Mossoro-Kpindé CD, Balekouzou A, Mavodé B, Andjingbopou Y. Seroprevalence of toxoplasmosis in women undergoing prenatal consultation at Bossembelé District Hospital in the Central African Republic in 2020. Rev Med Sante Trop. 2021;11:151-157.

[10]: BELAID A, BOUREDJI NE, MASTER'S MEMORANDUM. Toxoplasmosis in pregnant women: Seroprevalence and evaluation of risk factors. June 29, 2022.

[11]: Fersaoui D, Rahali S. IMMUNOLOGICAL MONITORING OF TOXOPLASMOSIS AND RUBEOLE IN PREGNANT WOMEN. Mémoire de Master. Academic year 2021-2022.

[12] : Hammaci L. Mémoire De fin d'études En vue de l'obtention du diplôme de Docteur en Pharmacie. Defended September 30, 2020.

[13]: Hamaichat M. Toxoplasmosis in pregnant women: Evaluation of seroprevalence, knowledge and preventive measures in the Guelmim region. Thesis presented and publicly defended on 24/07/2020.

 [14]: Akourim M. Perception and seroprevalence of Toxoplasmosis in pregnant women: Epidemiological survey in the Agadir-Inzegane region. Thesis presented and publicly defended on 17/06/2016.

[15] : Villard O, Cimon B, L'Ollivier C, et al. Help in the Choice of Automated or Semiautomated Immunoassays for Serological Diagnosis of Toxoplasmosis: Evaluation of Nine Immunoassays by the French National Reference Center for Toxoplasmosis. J Clin Microbiol. 2016;54(12):3034-3042.

 [16]: Robert-Gangneux F, Guegan H. Anti-Toxoplasma IgG assays: What performances for what purpose? A systematic review. Parasite (Paris, France). 2021; 28:39.

[17]: Teimouri A, Modarressi MH, Shojaee S, Mohebali M, Zouei N, Rezaian M, Keshavarz H. Detection of toxoplasma-specific immunoglobulin G in human sera: performance comparison of in house Dot-ELISA with ECLIA and ELISA. Springerplus. 2018 ;7(1) :372.

[18]: Dion S. Immune response and epidemiological markers in congenital toxoplasmosis. Sarra Dion. 2019.

Appendices

<u>Appendix</u> 1

Elecsys Toxo IgG; cobas e 411 (ECLIA) REF: 04618815119

Reagents - composition and concentrations

The reagent rackpack (M, R1, R2) is labelled TOXIGG.

M Streptavidin-coated microparticles, 1 vial (transparent cap), 6.5 mL: Streptavidin-coated microparticles 0.72 mg/mL, preservative

R1 Ag toxoplasmique~biotine, 1 vial (grey cap), 9 mL: T. gondi specific antigen (recombinant, E. Coli) biotinylated > 400 µg/L; TRIS buffer 50 mmol/L, pH 7.5; preservative

R2 Toxoplasmic ag~Ru(bpy) , 1 vial (black cap), 9 mL: ruthenium-labelled T. gondi specific antigen (recombinant, E. Coli) > 400 µg/L; TRIS buffer 50 mmol/L, pH 7.5; preservative

TOXIGG Cal1 Negative Calibrator 1 (white cap), 2 wells each containing 1.0 mL: human serum, non-reactive for anti-toxoplasmic IgG; buffer; preservative

TOXIGG Cal2 Positive Calibrator 2 (black cap), 2 wells each containing 1.0 mL: Human serum, reagent for antitoxoplasmic IgG-, approx. 100 IU/mL; buffer; preservative

Auxiliary equipment required

- Ref: 04618823190, PreciControl Toxo IgG, 16 x 1.0 mL

- Ref: 11732277122, Diluent Universal, 2 x 16 mL, sample diluent or 03183971122, Diluent Universal, 2 x 36 mL, sample diluent

- Ref 11776576322, CalSet Vials, 2 x 56 empty stoppered vials

- Usual laboratory equipment

- cobas e analyzer

Auxiliary equipment for cobas e 411 analyzer :

- Ref: 11662988122, ProCell, 6 x 380 mL, system buffer

- Ref: 11662970122, CleanCell, 6 x 380 mL washing solution for measuring cell

- Ref: 11930346122, Elecsys SysWash, 1 x 500 mL, washing solution additive

- Ref: 11933159001, SysClean Adapter, adapter for SysClean

- Ref: 11706802001, AssayCup, 60 x 60 reaction cuvettes

- Ref: 11706799001, AssayTip, 30 x 120 pipette tips

- Ref: 11800507001, Clean-Liner

Appendix 2

Platelia^{TM} Testline TOXO IgG REF: TgG096

- **Reagents (Figure 1)**

*Microtiter **plate**: antigen-sensitized, 12 x 8 wells in desiccant bag (1 pc).

*Negative control (standard 1) 0.1 U/ml: Solution containing no specific human antibodies, ready to use (1*2ml). *

Cut-off (standard 2) 6 IU/ml: Solution containing specific human antibodies, ready to use (1*3ml). *

Positive control (standard 3) 60 IU/ml: Solution containing specific human antibodies, ready for use (1*2ml).

*Sample diluent 5: Buffer with protein stabilizers, ready to use (1*105ml). *

TMB-Complete 2: Chromogenic substrate solution containing TMB/H202, ready to use (1*15ml).

*Wash solution: 20x concentrated buffer (1*75ml).

*Stop solution: Acid solution, ready to use (1*15ml).

- Reagent preparation :

*Dilute wash solution 1:20 (1 part solution and 19 parts distilled water); e.g. 75 ml concentrated wash solution + 1425 ml distilled water.

* Standards, conjugates and substrate (TMB-complete) are ready-to-use, no dilution required.

- Sample preparation :

*Mixing samples

*Dilute samples: serum/plasma 1:101 (10 µl + 1 ml)

- Semi-quantitative evaluation in positivity index :

*Leave the first well empty (white).

*Pipette 100ul of negative control into a well.

*Pipette 100ul of CUT-OFF (standard 2) into 2 wells.

*Pipette 100ul of positive control into a well.

*Pipette the diluted samples into the other wells.

* Cover the microplate with the lid and incubate at 37◦C for 60 minutes.

* Aspirate the contents of the wells and wash 5x with wash solution. Finally, press the microplate upside down onto absorbent paper to remove any remaining solution.

* Pipette 100 ul of conjugate into all wells except A1.
* Cover the microplate with the lid and incubate at 37◦C for 60 minutes.
* Aspirate the contents of the wells and wash 5x with wash solution. Finally, press the microplate upside down onto absorbent paper to remove any remaining solution.

* Pipette 100 ul of TMB-Complete into all wells. Avoid contamination.

* Cover the microplate with the lid and incubate at 37◦C for 20 minutes in the dark.

* Stop the reaction by adding 100 ul of the stop solution in the same order and intervals as the substrate was added. *Read the color intensity in the wells against the blank using a spectrophotometer set to 450 nm. Absorbance should be read within 30 minutes of stopping the reaction.

Appendix 3

Blot-line Toxoplasma IgG REF: TgGL20

+1 x 20 pieces BL STRIP: Sensitized strips of recombinant antigens

1x5 ml: Negative control: Solution containing no specific antibodies, ready to use

1x5 ml positive control: Solution containing specific antibodies, ready to use

2 x 20 ml conjugate: Solution containing (fraction of animal immunoglobulin to human IgG), ready to use

2 x 20 ml: Substrate solution: Buffer with BCIP and NBT, ready to use

1x 300 ml: Universal solution: Buffer for sample dilution and strip washing, ready to use.

2 pcs: Transparent adhesive film

+Sample preparation

Dilute well-mixed samples 1:51 with universal solution: 30 ul sample + 1.5 ml universal solution, mix well.

+Analysis procedure

1. Before use, remove all components from the kit box and allow them to equilibrate at room temperature for approximately 60 minutes. Mix well.

2. Pipette 2.5 ml of the universal solution into each well of the incubation tray. One well is required per test sample.

3. Use forceps to grasp the lower part of the strip not covered by the membrane, remove the buffer strip and place one strip in each well. The strip must be completely immersed in the universal solution. Incubate the BL strips at room temperature on a rocking shaker for 10 minutes. Immediately return the unused strips to the bag with desiccant and seal the bag.

4. Aspirate the universal solution from the wells.

5. Pipette 1.5 ml of the diluted samples into the wells and incubate on a rocker for 30 minutes. When using the Negative and Positive Controls, do not dilute them. They are ready to use. Alternatively, samples can be diluted directly in the wells. Pipette 1.5 ml of the universal solution into the wells with the wet strips. Then add 30 ul of sample to each well. This dilution method requires complete mixing of the well.

6. Aspirate diluted samples.

7. Wash strips with 1.5 ml of the universal solution for 3 x 5 minutes each time on a

shaker.

8. Pipette 1.5 ml of conjugate into each well and incubate at room temperature on a rocking shaker for 30 minutes.

9. Aspirate the conjugate.

10. Wash the strips with 1.5 ml of the universal solution 3 x 5minutes each time on a rocker shaker.

11. Pipette 1.5 ml of substrate solution into each well and incubate at room temperature on a rocking arm for 15 minutes.

12. Aspirate the substrate solution and wash each strip with 2 ml distilled water 2 x 5 minutes each time on a rocking shaker.

13. Remove the strips from the incubation tray and transfer them to the adhesive frames on the evaluation protocol. Allow strips to air-dry.

14. evaluate dried strips. For long-term storage, protect strips from light by covering them with a transparent self-adhesive sheet.

Appendix 4

Platelia™ Biorad TOXO IgG REF:72840

The test process comprises the following steps:

- **Step 1:** The samples to be studied and the calibrators are diluted 1:21 and then placed in the wells of the microplate. During this 1-hour incubation at 37°C, the anti-*T. gondii* IgG present in the sample binds to the T. gondi antigen bound to the microplate wells. Non-T. gondii-specific IgG and other serum proteins are removed by washing at the end of incubation.

- **Step 2:** The conjugate (peroxidase-labeled monoclonal antibody specific for human gamma chains) is deposited in all microplate wells. During this 1-hour incubation at 37°C, the labeled antibody binds to serum IgG that has reacted with the T. gondi antigen. Unbound conjugate is removed by washing at the end of incubation.

- **Step 3:** The presence of any complexes (*T. gondii* Ag, anti-*T. gondii* IgG, anti-IgG conjugate) formed is revealed by adding an enzymatic revelation solution to each cup.

- **Stage 4:** After incubation at room temperature (+18-30°C), the enzymatic reaction is stopped by adding a solution of 1N sulfuric acid. The optical density read at 450/620 nm is proportional to the amount of anti-*T. gondii* IgG present in the test sample. Optical density is converted to IU/ml using a standard reference range calibrated to WHO International Standard TOX-M.

Composition of the kit :

Labeling	Nature of reagents	Presentation
R4a Calibrator 6	**Calibrator 6 IU/ml**: Human serum reactive for anti-T. gondii IgG, and negative for HBsAg and for anti-HIV1, anti-HIV2 and anti-HCV antibodies Preservative: (0.098%) ProClin™ 300	1 x 0.75 ml
R4b Calibrator 60	**Calibrator 60 IU/ml**: Human serum reactive for anti-T. gondii IgG, and negative for HBsAg and for anti-HIV1, anti-HIV2 and anti-HCV antibodies Preservative: (0.098%) ProClin™ 300	1 x 0.75 ml
R4c Calibrator 240	**Calibrator 240 IU/ml**: Human serum reactive for anti-T. gondii IgG, and negative for HBsAg and anti-HIV1, anti-HIV2 and anti-HCV antibodies Preservative: (0.098%) ProClin™ 300	1 x 0.75 ml
R6 Conjugate (51X)	**Conjugate (51X):** Peroxidase-coupled mouse monoclonal anti-human gamma-chain antibody Preservative: (0.159%) ProClin™ 300	1 x 0.7 ml
R7 Thinner	Sample diluent and conjugate (ready-to-use): Tris-NaCl (pH 7.7), glycerol, 0.1% Tween® 20, phenol red Preservative: (0.148%) ProClin™ 300	1 x 100 ml
R9 Chromogen TMB	**Chromogen** (ready-to-use): 3,3',5,5' tetramethylbenzidine (< 0.1%), H_2O_2 (<1%)	1 x 28 ml
R10 Stopping Solution	**Stopping solution** (ready to use): 1N sulfuric acid solution	1 x 28 m

*** Reconstitution of reagents :**

 - R1: Allow to return to room temperature (+18-30°C) for 30 minutes before opening the sachet. Remove the frame and immediately replace any unused bars in the sachet, checking for the presence of desiccant. Carefully reseal the bag and store at +2-8°C.

- R2: Dilute solution R2 with distilled water to 1:20: 50 ml of R2 in 950 ml of distilled water. This produces a ready-to-use solution. Use 350 ml of diluted wash solution for a whole plate of 12 strips in manual washing.

- R3, R4a, R4b, R4c: Dilute 1:21 with Diluent (R7) (example: 300 µL R7 + 15 µL Calibrator).

- R6+R7: Conjugué R6 comes in 51-fold concentrated liquid form. Homogenize before use. Dilute 1:51 with Diluent (R7). For a full plate, dilute extemporaneously 0.5 ml Conjugate (R6) in 25 ml Diluent (R7). Divide volumes by 10 for one slide.

*** Procedure :**

1. Carefully plan the distribution and identification of calibrators and patient samples.

 2. Prepare dilute Wash Solution (R2) [Refer to chapter 7.2].

3. Remove the support frame and strips (R1) from the protective packaging [Refer to chapter 7.2].

4. In individually identified tubes, dilute calibrators R3, R4a, R4b, R4c and patient samples to be tested at 1/21 in Diluent (R7), i.e. 300 µl Diluent (R7) followed by 15 µl sample. Homogenize well (vortex).

5. Dispense 200µl of calibrators and diluted samples into each cup as follows:

	1	2	3	4	5	6	7	8	9	10	11	12
A	R3	S5	S13									
B	R4a	S6										
C	R4b	S7										
D	R4c	S8										
E	S1	S9										
F	S2	S10										
G	S3	S11										
H	S4	S12										

6.

Cover the microplate with adhesive film, pressing firmly over the entire surface to ensure a watertight seal. Then immediately incubate the microplate in a thermostated water bath or dry microplate incubator for 1 hour ± 5 minutes at 37°C ± 1°C.

7. Before the end of the first incubation, prepare the conjugate working solution (R6+R7).

8. At the end of the first incubation, remove the adhesive film, aspirate the contents of all cups into a contaminated waste container (containing sodium hypochlorite) and wash 4 times with 350 µl of Wash Solution (R2). Dry the strips by turning them over on a sheet of absorbent paper and tapping lightly to remove all the Wash Solution.

9. Immediately dispense 200 µl of conjugate working solution (R6+R7) into all wells. Shake gently before use.

10. Cover the microplate with new adhesive film, pressing firmly over the entire surface to ensure a watertight seal. Incubate the microplate in a thermostated water bath or dry microplate incubator for 1 hour ± 5 minutes at 37°C ± 1°C.

11. At the end of the second incubation, remove the adhesive film, aspirate the contents of all cups into a contaminated waste container (containing sodium hypochlorite) and wash 4 times with 350 µl of Wash Solution (R2). Dry the strips by turning them over on a sheet of absorbent paper and tapping lightly to remove all the Wash Solution.

12. Quickly dispense 200 µl of Chromogen (R9) into all wells, protected from bright light. Allow the reaction to develop in the dark for 30 ± 5 minutes at room temperature (+18-30°C). Do not use adhesive film during incubation.

13. Stop the enzymatic reaction by adding 100 µl of Stop Solution (R10) to each well. Follow the same sequence and rate of distribution as for the developer solution.

14. Carefully wipe off the underside of the plates. Read the optical density at 450/620 nm using a plate reader within 30 minutes of stopping the reaction. Always store plates in a dark place before reading.

15. Before transcribing the results, check that the reading matches the plate and sample distribution plan.

<u>Data collection form</u>

Date: .... Syslab number: ....

I.   Personal information

*Last name: .... First name: ....

*Age:...................... *Phone number:................

II.   Clinical information for pregnant women

*Number of pregnancies: ......

*Parity: Nullipare☐ Primipare☐ multipare☐

* Gestational age: 1st trimester ☐ 2nd trimester ☐ 3rd trimester ☐

III.   Serology

*Toxoplasmosis immune status :

IgG antibody titre by ECLIA: ....UI/ml

IgG antibody titre by Biorad ELISA: ....UI/ml

IgG antibody index by Testline ELISA: ....

IgG line blot result: negative ☐ doubtful ☐ positive ☐

<u>Summary</u>

Introduction :

Diagnosis of toxoplasmosis in pregnant women is compulsory, and mainly based on serology. Serology relies on several techniques based on the systematic detection of IgG and IgM. The aim of this study was to compare three serological techniques for the detection of anti-toxoplasmic IgG.

Materials and methods:

This is a cross-sectional study carried out in the Parasitology-Mycology laboratory of the Hôpital militaire principal d'instruction de Tunis during the period between January 23, 2023 and April 30, 2023. We studied IgG titres in 53 sera from pregnant women initially tested by the ECLIA technique (Elecsys® Toxo IgG), subdivided into three groups according to IgG levels. These sera were then re-tested by quantitative ELISA (Platelia™ Biorad), semi-quantitative ELISA (Platelia™ Testline) and Blot-line *Toxoplasma* IgG.

Results :

The mean age of our patients was 29 ± 3.9 years (extremes 22 and 40 years). Serologies were requested during their first pregnancies (72%), in primiparous women (51%) and in 67% during the first trimester. We compared 3 groups of sera: group 1 [30-300 IU/ml] (n=17), group 2 [300-1000 IU/ml) (n=19) and group 3 [> to 1000 IU/mL] (n= 17). ECLIA and quantitative and semi-quantitative ELISA showed complete agreement (p=1), but IgG titres by ECLIA were higher. Multiplication factors for ECLIA vs ELISA results were 2, 3 and 9 for groups 1, 2 and 3 respectively. On the other hand, an almost perfect agreement (P= 0.947) was found when comparing ECLIA and Western blot, given the presence of a doubtful case by Western blot with an IgG level of 39 IU/ml close to the positivity threshold (30 IU/ml) of ECLIA.

Conclusion:

Our study shows good agreement between the serological techniques used. ECLIA appears to be the most sensitive of the techniques studied. In addition, for titres close to the ECLIA positivity threshold, the use of a second confirmatory technique is recommended.

Key words: toxoplasmosis, ECLIA, ELISA, western blot, IgG.

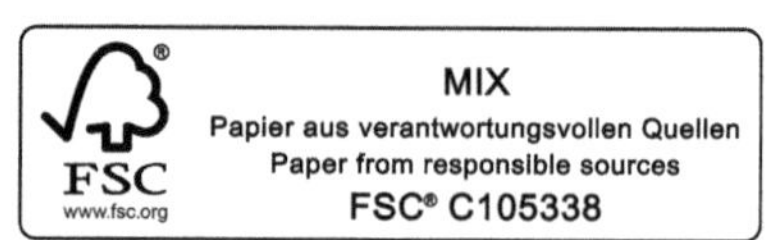

Printed by Books on Demand GmbH, Norderstedt / Germany